BED BUGS

The Proboscis Blood Sucker

Pierre Mouchette

Real Property Experts LLC
a Life Knowledge Publication

Copyright © 2019 by Pierre Mouchette
All rights reserved. No part of this publication may be reproduced or used in any manner without written permission of the Copyright Holder, except by a reviewer who may quote brief passages in a review.

First Edition: December 2020
Real Property Experts LLC
Web Address: https://www.rpe4u.com
Contact: publications@rpe4u.com

Note: This publication comes in a variety of formats, such as Paperbacks and Electronic Books (e-books). Some material included with the paperback versions of this book may not be included in e-books, and vice versa.

Disclaimer: This Real Property Experts LLC (RPE) publication provides information about the subject matter covered. The author and publisher of this content are not acting as licensed professionals in the presentation of covered material and are not qualified to give advice normally provided by professionals in the fields of expertise of this content, nor are they responsible for errors and omissions. The information and statements made, are for educational purposes and are not intended to replace a one-on-one relationship with a qualified attorney, accountant, tax professional, or other licensed professionals. You are solely responsible for the use of any content and hold Real Property Experts LLC, its' subsidiary's, and members harmless in any event or claim, demand, or damage, including reasonable attorneys' fees, asserted by any third party, or arising out of your use of, or conduct on, articles and/or products.

RPE writers provide applicable content and break down complex topics so they are easier to understand. Information given may not apply to your specific situation, and products or services recommended may not be a good fit for your application. While RPE strives to provide accurate up-to-date content, we cannot guarantee the accuracy and completeness of information provided. By using this content, you understand that all material is an expression of opinions and not professional advice.

RPE regularly updates articles, but it is possible that we may miss something. Use our content as a starting point before selecting to use and choose a service or product. The reader is advised to keep up to date on activities in their locale by consulting with the appropriate licensed professionals for decisions that could affect them.

PREFACE

Among all possible pest infestations, bed bugs present themselves as one of the most problematic, both in terms of health and in terms of solution. Yet this infestation is also one of the most common! According to the Centers for Disease Control and Prevention, bed bugs can cause serious health hazards. In addition to the discomfort and itching caused by their bites (the hollow tubes they use to pierce your skin and suck your blood contain a powerful but temporary painkiller), you will not feel their handiwork until hours later, when you can develop skin rashes, allergic symptoms, and even psychological problems. Bed bugs are not known to transmit any disease pathogens!

For comments on this publication please write to us at REAL PROPERTY EXPERTS LLC.

Pierre Mouchette, author

SPECIAL FEATURES

This book comes with a Website
(https://www.synchronicity-investor.com)

THE SYNCHRONICITY INVESTOR website provides world class solutions for all. No matter if you are an individual, a small business owner, or a decision maker at a conglomerate, THE SYNCHRONICITY INVESTOR is committed to providing you with the information that you need to make informed decisions. We encourage you to think of THE SYNCHRONICITY INVESTOR as your go to source for knowledgeable information. Additionally, on the website you can:

- Keep up to date - when there are important changes to our publications, we will post updates on-line.

- Publications - the website contains hundreds of articles on Real Estate, everyday Life, and the Environment, written by Pierre Mouchette and available for free. There you will find more Books, Booklets, How-to-Articles, Guides and much, much more.

Contents

Bed Bug FAQ

✓ Bed Bugs get their name from the fact that they are usually found near beds.

✓ Bed Bugs can mature in about 35 days.

✓ Bed bugs cannot climb smooth surfaces.

✓ In temperatures over 110 degrees Fahrenheit, bed bugs cannot live for more than three or four hours.

✓ Bed Bugs can go without a meal for more than a year.

✓ Bed Bugs do not limit themselves to hiding in beds. Some bed bugs will travel up to 100 feet in search of a host, but on average, most bed bugs will not travel more than 30 feet. Bed bugs can only move about 3 to 4 feet per minute.

✓ After Bed Bugs feed, they retreat to their hiding place for days or even weeks before coming back out. This can make detection difficult until the infestation is well established.

Pest control professionals should be consulted as early as possible to identify and control a potential infestation.

- 7 -

Chapter 1   BED BUGS

What Are Bed Bugs?

Bed bugs are parasites that belong to the **'cimicidae family.'** They are small, oval, brownish insects that feed exclusively on blood. While there are quite a few parasites of the cimicid family that feeds on animal blood, the **'cimex lectularius,'** prefers to feed on human blood.

Although bed bugs are believed to be more active during the night, they are not nocturnal. Bed bugs excel at hiding in dark, soft places and crevices. This makes the mattress an ideal spot for them to settle, hence the name bed bug. Bed bugs cannot fly, but they can move over floors, walls, and ceilings.

Scientific Classification of Bed Bugs

Kingdom

Animalia - animals are multicellular eukaryotic organisms that form the biological kingdom Animalia. With few exceptions, animals consume organic material, breathe oxygen, can move, can reproduce sexually, and grow from a hollow sphere of cells, the blastula, during embryonic development.

Phylum

Arthropoda - An invertebrate animal having an exoskeleton (external skeleton), a segmented body, and paired jointed appendages.

Class

Insecta - insects have a chitinous exoskeleton, a three-part body (head, thorax, and abdomen), three pairs of jointed legs, compound eyes and one pair of antennae.

Order

Hemiptera - These are true bugs, an order of insects comprising some 50,000 to 80,000 species of groups such as the cicadas, aphids, planthoppers, leafhoppers, and shield bugs.

Family
Cimicidae - a family of small parasitic insects that feed exclusively on the blood of warm-blooded animals

Genus
Cimex - a genus of insects in the family Cimicidae. Cimex species are ectoparasites that typically feed on the blood of birds and mammals. Two species, Cimex lectularius and Cimex hemipterus, are known as bed bugs and frequently feed on humans, although other species may parasitize humans opportunistically.

The above classification information was obtained from **Wikipedia, the free encyclopedia.**

Identifying Bed Bugs

Characteristics such as color, shape and size will help you to distinguish bed bugs from other insects. The actual size of bed bugs can vary, depending on their life stage and age. The following is a general bed bug size comparison at each stage:

Eggs are tiny, about the size of a pin head (1 mm)

- 1st stage nymph (1.5 mm).

- 2nd stage nymph (2 mm).

- 3rd stage nymph (2.5 mm).

- 4th stage nymph (3 mm), about the size of a sesame seed.

- 5th stage nymph (4.5 mm).

- Adult bed bugs (5-7 mm or 3/16-1/4 inch), about the size of an apple seed.

The life cycle of a bed bug includes multiple nymphal stages, with the insect **'blood feeding'** between each nymphal stage. Bed bugs typically mature in two to six weeks (depending on environmental temperature and availability of blood meal hosts). Adults can survive for six months to a year without blood; however, the females must have a blood meal in order to reproduce. Ideal temperature for bed bug propagation is above 70°F. Considering a single female can lay between 200 and 500 eggs in a lifetime even a single bed bug sighting should be taken seriously to help curtail the reproductive cycle of these insects.

In general, adult bed bugs are:

- About the size of an apple seed.

- Flat, oval-shaped, and reddish-brown (if not blood fed recently).

- Balloon-like and bright red (if blood fed recently).

- Produce a foul, somewhat musty odor.

- Not known to jump or fly, but crawl instead.

- Unlikely to live on human hosts but come out from their hiding spots to blood feed.

Bed Bug Anatomy

The following is a detailed description of the parts of an adult bed bug's body:

- Head - they have a short broad head that attaches to the thorax.

- Proboscis - a small tube located under the mouth that elongates when the bed bug is ready to feed. A bed bug draws about 0.0055 milliliters of blood per bite.

- Eyes - bed bugs have compound eyes, in which a single large eye is made up of many repeating units called ommatidia.

- Antennae - the bed bugs sensors have four segments each and are about half its body length. These sensors guide the bed bugs to their host.

- Wing Pads - adults are equipped with vestigial wings (underdeveloped), and they cannot fly.

- Abdomen - has 11-segments that expand as the bed bug gouges itself with blood during feeding. The male has a pointed tip abdomen and the female a rounded tip.

- Setae - tiny sensory structures covering the abdomen (they look like mini-hairs).

- Thorax - the body segment where the legs are attached, enabling the bed bug to move.

- Legs - they have six legs that are adapted for crawling. Their claws are used for gripping rough surfaces as well as the host (you) when feeding.

Chapter 2   BED BUG BITES

Bed Bugs Hide During the Day and Feed at Night

To track their food source, bed bugs follow the carbon dioxide we exhale. To increase bite precision, they also track the warmth our bodies give off. After locating a food source, the bug crawls up to the skin and commences feeding.

How Do Bed Bugs Feed?

Bed bugs usually bite people at night while they are sleeping. The bed bug pierces the skin with its elongated beak (proboscis) through which it withdraws blood. This engorgement takes about three to ten minutes, yet the victim seldom knows they are being bitten. They continue to draw blood from the host until they are gorged.

Why You Do Not Feel the Bite

When drawing blood, this bug injects saliva right into the spot where the blood is being drawn. The saliva or the proteins in it called sialomes (contains an anesthetic), acts as a painkiller, but also irritates the skin and it is this irritation that causes you to scratch.

Note: there are also other proteins in bed bug saliva that dilate the blood vessel (vasodilators), and anti-clotting agents (anticoagulants), which overcome the body's natural defenses that stop bleeding. This allows for steady blood flow when bed bugs are feeding.

Do Bed Bug Bites Spread If You Scratch Them?

Bedbugs do bite, and their bites can be discomforting. Although people react differently to the bite, people bitten by the bugs may find themselves scratching the bitten spot. In severe cases, rashes might develop, and incessant scratching might result in a welt. These bites will not spread because they are non-contagious.

Treatment for Bed Bug Bites

In most cases, bedbug bites get better within one to two weeks. To relieve symptoms, it may help to:

- Apply anti-itch cream or calamine lotion to bites.

- Take an oral antihistamine to reduce itching and burning.

- Use an over-the-counter pain reliever to relieve swelling and pain.

In rare cases, bed bug bites can cause allergic reactions. If your child gets bit, talk to your child's doctor or pharmacist before using topical steroid creams or oral antihistamines to treat the bites. Some medications may not be safe for babies or young children. **If signs or symptoms of a serious allergic reaction develop, go to a walk-in center, or call 911.**

Sometimes, bed bug bites can cause an infection known as cellulitis. To reduce the risk of infection, wash the bites with soap and water and try not to scratch them.

Your Pets

Bedbugs do not just bite humans. They can also feed on family pets. If you have a pet who has been bitten by bed bugs, the bites will likely get better on their own. But in some cases, they might become infected. Make an appointment with a veterinarian if you suspect your pet has an infected bite.

What Are Symptoms of a Bed Bug Infestation?

The most common symptoms are:

- Blood stains on sheets or pillowcases.

- Morning itching.

- Red bites with a swollen area around a darker color in the center.

- Small swollen areas where there is more than one bite, or a group of bites.

- Hives and blisters where the bites are.

- Bed bug excrement (little black dot and stains) on the bed, bed linen or walls.

- Eggshells or shed skins (tiny specks of ivory material) in areas where bed bugs hide.

- A musty odor from the bugs' scent glands.

Chapter 3   BED BUG INFECTION and CONTROL

Bed Bug Control

Bed bugs are a challenging pest to control. They hide in the tiniest of places so when found or suspected, a professional pest exterminator should be obtained. Experience pest control operators know what to do and how to do it. Getting an inspection and treatment Is essential. All excess clutter should be removed. Infested mattresses and box springs should be immediately removed from the premises. Adjoining housing must be inspected to determine if the bugs have traveled.

Where Are Suspect Hiding Places for Bed Bugs?

If you suspect there are bedbugs in your home, look for signs in:

- mattresses
- box springs
- bed frames
- headboards
- pillows and bedding
- cracks or seams of furniture
- carpeting around baseboards
- spaces behind light switches and electrical outlet plates
- curtains
- clothes
- shoes

Once bed bugs are introduced to an environment they rapidly spread from room to room through a building. **'The level of cleanliness of the house or building has nothing to do with bed bug infestation.'** If they have a warm body, they will proliferate.

Do Bed Bugs Fly?

Although they have wings, bed bugs cannot fly. They cannot jump either, so their primary means of motion is to crawl. Bed

Bugs are excellent at hitching a ride from one location to another. They crawl into luggage, shopping bags and any number of stored goods, and are easily transported. If you are unfortunate enough to find bed bugs in your home, it is likely that you brought them in from somewhere else.

How Do Bed Bugs Travel?

These bugs can be brought into your home via visitors, luggage, used furniture, used beds, clothing, etc. They are not picky about where and when they catch a ride and do not necessarily have a preferred mode of transportation. **'Bed bugs do not have a preference between a spotless space or a filthy environment. If they have access to a food source, they can live anywhere.'**

Did you know that bed bugs can hide and be transferred from one place to another in your books, bags, and belongings? You might spot them hiding out in:

- **Books** - if you have noticed black spots on the edge of a book, it may be bed bugs. Due to their small size, bed bugs can fit into several different parts of a book. This includes the binding, fore-edge, and protective covering. Bed bugs can be found in or on books or magazines that are placed near resting areas.
Determine if bed bugs are hiding in your books. To avoid migration, keep a vacuum close by. Seal infested books within a plastic bag immediately, and put lemongrass, or clove in the bag. Keep books in the plastic bag for three weeks. Or contact a pest management professional. A pest control specialist can help remove them and inspect other areas to which bed bugs could have migrated.

- **Luggage** - when traveling, bed bugs might hitch a ride on your luggage. If bed bugs are not detected before you arrive at your destination, you risk spreading the infestation. Use a flashlight to check all areas of your bag, including pockets and seams. If you find bed bugs in your luggage, vacuuming with a crevice tool attachment can move them into the vacuum bag. This will not kill the bugs, but it may contain them within the vacuum bag. When emptying the bag, it is important that you remove all bed bugs. If left inside the bag, they could escape. It may be best to seal the vacuum bag in a plastic bag and put lemongrass, or clove in the bag. Dispose of the plastic bag in a sealed garbage can as far away from the house as possible. Your luggage should be cleaned by professionals to ensure proper extermination.

- **Shoes** - do you have a closet full of barely worn shoes? In shoes, bed bugs can hide under soles, between fabrics and in crevices. Before inspecting the shoe, make sure you wear protective gloves as you will need to be hands-on. Examine all materials, layers, laces, zippers, and mesh. If you find bed bugs or suspect their presence, move shoes into a plastic bag or container and put lemongrass, or clove in the container or call a pest management professional. These specialists can provide proper instructions on how to salvage your shoes and help ensure the infestation does not spread.

- Electronics - yes, bed bugs can find their way into electronics with small openings. To inspect your devices, use a magnifying glass and make sure you are aware of the common bed bug signs. If you spot any bed bugs, you may not want to take matters into your own hand. Attempting any do-it-yourself solutions can put both you and your electronics at risk. Additionally, you may worsen your chances of safely removing them from your device. As a safety precaution, call in help from a pest management professional.

How Bed Bugs Become an Infestation?

Every day, bed bugs can lay between 1 and 12 eggs, and anywhere from 200 and 500 eggs in a lifetime. Those numbers speak for themselves if you are wondering how long it takes to get an infestation of bed bugs. Bed bugs need to take blood meals from warm-blooded hosts, typically humans to survive, and they will hide near their sources until ready to feed. After feeding, bed bugs head back to their hidden locations to digest and mate. Bed bugs are focused on feeding and breeding and will invade and multiply at lightning speed as a result.

Get Rid of Bed Bugs Naturally

You may be interested in taking a natural approach for the following reasons:

- It is low-cost (maybe even free).

- You can act right away.

- You avoid toxic chemicals that an exterminator uses.

Note: most solutions utilize things you already have in the house, but if you do need to go out and purchase something, it will be relatively inexpensive. Commercially available repellents can get rid of bed bugs, but they can cause damage to your health.

GENERAL

- **Baking Soda** - it will suck the moisture out of bed bugs' bodies. To use this powder, spread it wherever you find the bugs, including cracks and crevices. Be sure to vacuum and reapply every few days.

- **Double-sided Tape** - wrap along the circumference of the bedposts near the floor. As the bugs try to climb up into the bed, they will get stuck.

- **Rubbing Alcohol** - pour it in a SPRAY BOTTLE and spritz away. The alcohol will kill bugs on contact.

- **Scented Dryer Sheets** - the smell from the dryer sheets can repel the insects and even encourage them to seek out other spots to inhabit. However, this is a temporary solution because they will just find a more hospitable place in the home to hang out.

- **Vacuum** - use the suction from your vacuum cleaner and a powerful hose attachment. You should probably vacuum at least every few days while battling an infestation. Be thorough and use the vacuum on the mattress, bedding, and soft furniture like sofas and cushy chairs. When you have completed the vacuuming, discard the vacuum bag outside, as far away from your home as possible. Steam clean all of those places the vacuum cannot reach, if possible. The heat will kill the bedbugs and their eggs, and they will die when exposed to temperatures exceeding 140 degrees Fahrenheit.

- **Washing all Clothes and Bedding** - check labels to verify the fabrics can tolerate hot water and tumble drying. Then wash everything that has been exposed. The combination of hot water and dryer heat will help kill off bed bugs.

HERBAL

- **Bean Leaves** - they work as a natural flypaper to trap insects, including bed bugs. Back in 1943, researchers discovered that the microscopic hairs on the leaves worked to both entangle and impale bed bug limbs. Put the leaves on the floor of any room with these unwanted inhabitants.

- **Beauveria Bassiana** - this is a parasitic fungus that feeds on insects. It ruthlessly attacks bed bugs, rendering them infertile, immobile, and unable to feed.

- **Black Walnut Tea** - this variety of tea is a natural insect repellent. To employ this strategy, simply take your used tea bags and put them in areas that are infested with the bugs. Place them around the house, and in every nook, cranny, and corner you can think of.

- **Cayenne Pepper** - when mixed with other natural items like ginger and oregano, cayenne pepper kills a bed bug on contact. To make this solution: Mix one teaspoon each of cayenne pepper, ground ginger, and oregano oil; strain the ingredients and add to a SPRAY BOTTLE filled with water; SPRAY!

- **Clove** - acts the same way as lemongrass. If you are not a fan of how lemongrass smells, opt for cloves and clove oil instead. You can even put clove oil on mattresses and pillows to ward bed bugs off.

- **Indian Lilac** - the leaves have a similar effect to other plant-based, herbal remedies. You can crush the leaves and spread them about or alternatively, boil the leaves, strain the solution, and add it to your bath water. The result is that bed bugs will no longer snack on you! This technique can also be used for closet and clothes infestations. SPRAY the solution in closets, on sofas, and around the home to repel bed bugs.

- **Lavender** - the smell of lavender makes a bed bug feel nauseous and can even lead to their death. Most people find the scent quite pleasant. Triple the effectiveness of this solution by washing items with lavender soap, spraying diluted essential oils, and spreading leaves over affected areas.

- **Lemongrass (citronella)** - unlike some of the other natural solutions that only repel the insects, lemongrass kills them. The acid levels kill the bugs and their eggs. Additionally, they hate the smell, so it does also serve as a repellent.

- **Mint Leaves** - are a preventive measure. If you place crushed leaves around entry points, it will dissuade bed bugs from coming into your home. They are also safe to use in your closet and directly on your mattress.

- **Orange Oil** - essential oils of orange contain d-limonene which is classified as an insecticide. This is a nerve toxin which kills bugs and insects within minutes of contact. Make a SPRAY solution by mixing 1 cup of compost tea, 1 ounce of blackstrap molasses and 2 ounces of orange essential oil in 4 liters of water. Mix all this together well and SPRAY in the affected areas.

- **Peppermint Leaves** - the leaves have the same effect as lavender oil and leaves. Utilize the same strategies and do not forget to regularly vacuum up old leaves and replace them with fresh versions until the infestation is gone.

- **Pyrethrum** - this extract is derived from Chrysanthemums. The Chrysanthemum (mum) is a bright flower that can be found in a variety of colors. It also works as a natural killer by attacking the bed bugs nervous system.

- **Sweet Flag** - a plant found mostly in wetlands is also an effective insect repellent. The herbal version comes in a packet that you can mix into a solution and SPRAY around the house.

- **Tea Tree Oil** - a fresh-smelling essential oil that has antimicrobial properties. It kills bacteria and fungi and neutralizes viruses on contact. It works on bed bugs by suffocating them as the oil works its way into their system. However, it is most effective when used

undiluted.
Note: an undiluted version is not safe for humans. To make the diluted formula, place about 20 drops of oil in A SPRAY BOTTLE filled with water.

- **Thyme** - if you tie a slick of thyme with a cloth, and then burn it near infested areas, the bugs will look for friendlier quarters. As always, practice fire safety.

Get Rid of Bed Bugs Mechanically

Bed Bug Heat Treatment Options

These are eco-friendly means to get rid of bed bugs. Bed bugs and their eggs are killed at 114F. Higher temperatures are used on the surface to make sure that enough heat penetrates any crack where bed bugs may be hiding.

- **Use Heat from A Hair Dryer** - heat can be safely applied to areas such as a mattress seam with a hair dryer on the high heat setting. Hold the hair dryer for 10 seconds on each spot to ensure that the proper amount of heat is applied. This method works well along mattress and box spring seams, around the headboard and along wall baseboards.

- **Handheld Steamer** - a professional grade steamer will product heat at about 200+ degrees, a level that will kill all bed bugs and eggs that meet the steam. This is a very safe and effective method. Differences between steam models include the amount of water they can hold and the ability to adjust the steam pressure.

- 27 -

AFTERWORD

- 28 -

Thank you for reading

BED BUG – The Proboscis Blood Sucker

We hope you enjoyed this Life Knowledge Publication

Thank you again valued reader,
and we hope to meet you again on another book.

ABOUT THE AUTHOR

Pierre Mouchette is the Founder and CEO of Real Property Experts LLC. He is a graduate of New York University, with a Master's in Business Administration, a Certificate in Real Estate Law - Fairfield University - CT, Graduate of the Realtors Institute - CT, and held licensing as a Real Estate Broker, and a Mortgage Broker.

Pierre is currently authoring Books, Booklets, How-to-Articles, and Guides in retirement. Pierre has an extensive background in real estate investment, business management and sales, supplemented by decades of hands-on-experience in building systems engineering, development, evaluation, and assorted analytical engineering studies.

Using background knowledge and experience, Pierre launched Real Property Experts in 2013 to help simplify real estate investing by connecting investors through innovative technology. In 2018, Pierre created THE SYNCHRONICITY INVESTOR a real estate website to facilitate providing world-class solutions for real estate investors and investment businesses.

Life Knowledge Publications

By Pierre Mouchette

ARACHNIDS, BUGS, INSECTS and REPTILES

The North American House Dust Mite

STINK BUGS aka SHIELD BUGS – The Stinky Insect

SPIDERS – The Venomous Eight -Legged PREDATOR

SNAKES – A Dubious Friend

FUNGUS GNATS – The Minute Flying Pests

CENTIPEDE – The Multi-Legged Venomous MONSTER

ANTS – A Diverse Society of Superorganisms

MOSQUITOES – The Midget Blood Suckers

ANIMALS

PETS – A Symbiotic Relationship Between Humans and Animals

BED BUGS – The Proboscis Blood Sucker

SKUNK – The American Polecat

DOGS – Responsibly Feeding Our Best Friends